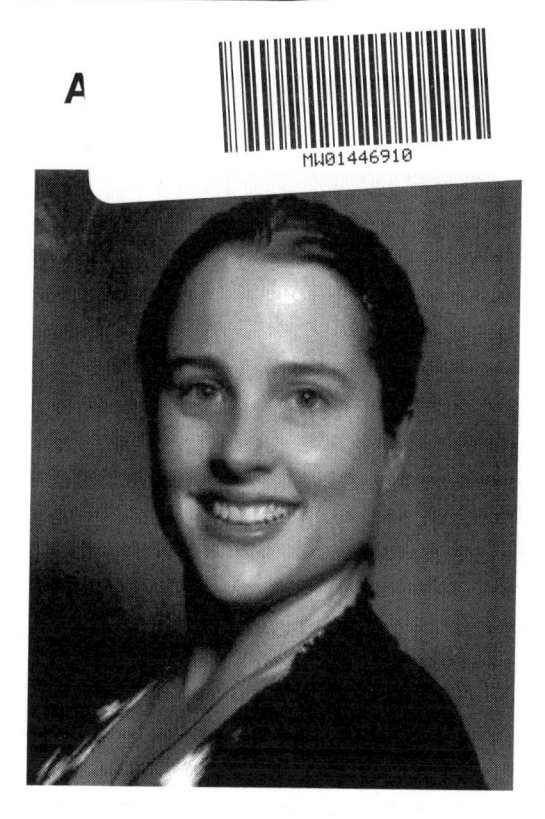

Thanks so much for purchasing my new book "Water Fasting For Wellness". My name is Jennifer Matthews and I go by the tagline "Naturopath Jen", because I am in fact a qualified Naturopath. I own the websites "Ask Naturopath Jen", "Low Carb Keto Living", "Passive Income Entrepreneur" and "Save On A Budget" which cover 2 of my greatest passions in life (health and wealth).

I have numerous facebook groups, a twitter account and even google plus. I am also in the process of building up "The Wellness Empire" as a hub for all of my websites.

ABOUT THE BOOK

If you are struggling with that stubborn body fat, you are wanting a good detox or you are suffering from an illness that just doesn't seem to be getting better, then water fasting may be just for you.

I wrote this book to inform you about the amazing benefits associated with water fasting. It has been used extensively in the treatment of autoimmune diseases, cardiovascular disease (especially hypertension) and not to mention to ward off the side effects of cancer treatments.

But of course one of the most amazing benefits is its ability to help you shift that last bit of excess weight, help clear up your skin and increase your longevity.

If you are not yet convinced that water fasting is something that you would like to try, then read on and I hope that by the end you may decide that it is something you can do. I have done it myself - and you can too...

However, don't worry... If a Water Fast seems too extreme to start off with, I have also included some information on 2 other forms of fasting - intermittent fasting and bone broth fasting.

And, if Water Fasting seems too easy and you are wanting results even quicker then you can try the "Dry Fast". However, remember that this is very extreme and should be done under the supervision of a practitioner. All in all, I think a Water Fast is your best bet.

Within this book I have answered 16 of the most common questions asked about fasting and have gone in depth on how to prepare for a fast, how to complete the fast and how to break the fast. Let me give you a tip - It is not just about the food. There is a lot of mindset work that needs to also be done. I go into the benefits of meditation during the fast, as well as the importance of keeping active.

DISCLAIMER

Please note that the information given in this book is for informational purposes only and is not intended to replace the advice of your health practitioner. If you experience symptoms that you are concerned with please refer to your practitioner for further information...

CONTENTS

ABOUT THE AUTHOR...1
ABOUT THE BOOK..2
DISCLAIMER..3
CONTENTS...4
Chapter 1 – Introduction to Fasting...5
Chapter 2 – History of Fasting..7
Chapter 3 – Benefits of Fasting - Introduction....................11
Chapter 4 – Benefits of Fasting – Brain Health...................13
Chapter 5 – Benefits of Fasting – Immune System/Cancer.......23
Chapter 6 – Benefits of Fasting – Fat Loss...........................27
Chapter 7 – Benefits of Fasting – Other................................31
Chapter 8 – Case Studies – Autoimmune Disease..............33
Chapter 9 – Case Studies – Cancer...37
Chapter 10 – Deciding If A Fast Is Right For You...............39
Chapter 11 – Preparing For A Water Fast............................43
Chapter 12 – Completing The Water Fast............................51
Chapter 13 – Exiting The Water Fast....................................55
Chapter 14 – Summary Of The 13 Steps To A Successful Water Fast..57
Chapter 15 – Common Fasting Questions Answered........59
Chapter 16 – Other Fasting Protocols...................................69
Chapter 17 – Conclusion...81
Chapter 18 – References - Scientific......................................83
Chapter 19 – References - Websites......................................85

Chapter 1 – Introduction to Fasting

What Is Fasting?

Fasting is a natural process that occurs within all of us on a daily basis – whether we try to or not. Fasting is basically the abstinence from food and caloric beverages, and believe it or not every night when we are sleeping we are actually in a fasted state.

There are many different types of fasts, which I will go into a little later in the book and they can range in effectiveness, efficiency and difficulty. They can range from the "Water Only" fast (covered in great detail in this book) where you consume nothing but pure water for a specified period of time all the way through to the "Intermittent Fast" which allows you to eat but only within a set number of hours throughout the day (broken down briefly in Chapter 11).

Which fasting regime you pick will be dependent on your personal goal, how quickly you are wanting to reach that goal and how strict you are willing to be with yourself. For instance, if you have an autoimmune disease or an illness that you are really wanting to correct as quickly as possible because it is becoming too hard to handle then a water fast is probably what you are looking for. Yes, it is difficult for the first couple of days but once the ketones kick in and you start burning fat, the cravings will disappear and you will no longer feel like eating. It is a very spiritual form of fasting that really allows you to get in touch with your own body.

Water fasting allows you to use the energy that you normally would for digestion to cleanse the body of accumulated toxins and heal any organs or tissues that are ill.

As the fast progresses the body will begin to consume everything that is not essential for the normal bodily functions, including bacteria, viruses, tumors, waste products, fluid buildup around the joints and even to remove stored fat.

When we look at the history and evolution of fasting (discussed next...) you will begin to realize that humans are actually designed to fast.

Chapter 2 – History of Fasting

If you look back to evolution and to the caveman day (if that is something that you believe in) then you will see that fasting is something they did on a daily if not weekly basis. They did not have an unlimited supply of food on hand like we do in today's society nor did they have a 7-11 down the street that they could go to and pick up a doughnut and slushy. The food that they had was purely what they could either hunt or gather and this meant they could go an unknown period of time without eating.

This meant that their bodies had to adapt to surviving on the fuel that they did have – which was basically ketones. Their bodies started to utilize the fatty acids stored in their fat cells and convert them into ketones to use for energy. Although this concept is unknown to most of us because we are constantly bombarding our bodies with endless supplies of food it is actually a natural process that gives our body the break and trains it to survive in times when food is scarce.

Pretty much every mammal on earth will fast during periods of stress or illness. Do you ever wonder why when you are ill you do not feel like eating? This is the body's natural way of healing.

During times of stress or sickness your body will recognize that it needs to rest, seek balance and conserve energy during these times. Digestion in itself is a very energy consuming task and so by fasting and abstaining from caloric beverages and foods during this period it gives the systems within your body the time to recover from whatever is happening.

Now, when we talk about the history of fasting we would be remiss to not mention the greatest historians of our time (especially in the wellness area), known as Hippocrates, Plato, Socrates, Aristotle and even Galen. Paracelsus who has been praised as one of three fathers of western medicine has labelled fasting as being the greatest remedy for healing.

Then of course you have to look at the many religions that practice fasting on a regular basis, such as:

Buddhists

The Buddhist fast in order to practice self-control and self-discipline. They believe in adopting a fast on certain days of the year (predominantly full moons) so as to give up food for those less fortunate than them.

This fasting requires not being able to eat after noon and it is a practice that is often done during times of intensive meditation, such as retreats.

Catholics

When it comes to fasting and the Roman Catholics they are only required to fast on ash Wednesday, Good Friday and all the Fridays of lent (40 day prep leading up to Easter) If they are over 14 years of age. In this time they must abstain from eating meat and items made from meat.

In some instances they are also required to abstain from meat on every Friday of the year.

Orthodox

Within the Orthodox Church, fasting is an absolutely critical element. They believe that as long as you are in the church you are required to fast but they leave it up to the individual as to the intensity of the fast.

Fasting days for all Orthodox Christians are every Wednesday and Friday throughout the year (except for the fast free days), Great Lent, Nativity Fast, Apostles Fast, Dormition Fast and a few special days. The calendar of fasting for the Orthodox is very complex and far too complicated to go into in detail.

Hindu's

Within the Hindu faith, fasting is classified as a very important aspect. Hindus will observe the fast in the name of a particular God every once, twice or more times a week. Depending on the deity they are wanting to please they will fast on that particular day.

For instance, for Lord Shiva somebody may choose to fast on Mondays, for Lord Dattatreya somebody may choose to fast on Thursdays and for Lord Hanuman somebody may choose to fast on Saturdays. There does not seem to be a fasting day for Wednesdays. On top of that they have a number of other religious fasting days such as Chaturthi and Gokulashtami (amongst others).

Their fasting involves fasting until the afternoon on water and then drinking fruit juice or one or two fruits. They allow you to break the fast in the evening after sunset. Timing for the fast is either from sunrise to sunset or a full 24 hour fast from 12am one day to 12am the next.

To the Hindu's it is a very spiritual process and they believe that if your body undergoes suffering (as in abstaining from food) then your sins will be lessened. They also believe that if you fast on a particular day, that deity will be happy with you and will lessen your sufferings. It is a very interesting practice.

Jews

When the Jews fast it means that they completely abstain from all foods and drink (including water). Jews will generally fast 6 days of the year, with Yom Kippur being the most important Jewish day of the year and which requires all Jews to participate in a fast (as long as they are above the bar mitzvah age). The only people that are exempt from fasting on this day are the ill or the frail.

Tisha B'Av is the other major fasting day for the Jews, which is a day that is remembered from 2500 years ago where the Babylonians destroyed the holy temple in Jerusalem and where the Romans destroyed the second holy temple in Jerusalem 2000 years ago.

Within the Jewish community there are a number of minor fasts which take place and they are also undertaken in the occurrence of a marriage.

There are three main reasons why Jews fast:

- For the purpose of achieving atonement and avert catastrophe;
- Commemorative Mourning; and
- Commemorative Gratitude.

Mormons

The Mormons will skip breakfast and lunch on the first Sunday of every month. In traditional Mormon churches the sum of money that would have been spent on those two meals is given to the bishop for any member that may be struggling. Although they don't recommend fasting for extended periods of time, one 24 hour fast a month is generally accepted.

They believe that fasting can be used alongside prayer when trying to discover answers to questions and some Mormons actually fast during especially stressful situations when they are trying to achieve clarity.

Muslims

You have probably heard of the spiritual practice known as "Ramadan". This is a fasting regime which is carried out by the Muslim community for a total of 30 days, once a year. It is a time of spiritual reflection, improvement and an increased devotion and worship.

For 30 days, all Muslims over the age of Puberty (as long as they are not ill or have no disabilities or illnesses). They do have exemptions however for those that are travelling, menstruating, have a serious illness, are pregnant or are breastfeeding.

They are required to fast between sunrise and sunset and the fast is broken with a few dates followed by a banquet style meal of appetizers, salads, main meat dishes and desserts.

Summary:

Fasting is a ritual that has been a necessary part of spirituality for thousands of years and thankfully research is now starting to recognize the benefits of such fasts. Many of the religions practice intermittent fasting where they are still allowed to eat and some require full water fasting.

Chapter 3 – Benefits of Fasting - Introduction

In recent years fasting has begun to be recognized as a therapeutic therapy for a multitude of conditions and for overall longevity. More and more research is being carried out (mostly in rodents) demonstrating these benefits.

However fasting provides not only physiological benefits but spiritual and mental benefits as well. Prior to going into the physiological benefits I think it is pertinent to list some of the spiritual and mental benefits you may experience.

Spiritual/Mental Benefits

Fasting is known to improve mental clarity and focus and therefore it can be used as a tool to give you a greater sense of freedom, flexibility and the level of energy you need to achieve those goals you have set for yourself.

Many people who fast find it helpful to do so at a time when they are requiring the extra energy to meet a major deadline or project. If you are in the process of completing something that requires you to be extra creative then fasting is a great way of going about it. In fact, artists do it all the time.

However, I must warn you. If it is your first time doing a water fast it is not a good idea to do it right before a major event as it takes a little while to begin to experience these effects.

Emotionally you may find that your depression lifts and you start to see things in a whole new light. Things may become clearer and more focused and you may start to believe that obstacles you once thought were too big now seem like minute obstacles that you can pass.

Of course another benefit of fasting is the ability to really connect with your spiritual side. It allows you to take your focus inwards and delve into who you really are and what your purpose is. Without the continual addition of heavy foods in your system your body will start to take on a lighter feeling.

During fasting, it is a great time to integrate some meditation or prayer into your day. People often find that during a fast meditation is easier and things are a lot clearer.

Physiological Benefits

Although there are numerous types of fasting such as intermittent fasting, dry fasting, bone broth fasting, juice fasting and of course water fasting, consuming only water for a set period of time will not only produce the results in the quickest amount of time with what I suspect the least amount of side effects. Out of all of the fasting types it provides the quickest detox and the strongest therapeutic effect.

Water Fasting is used for many common conditions in today's society such as autoimmune diseases, brain health, skin disorders and in particular immune health and cancer prevention. There have been a multitude of studies done on intermittent fasting with very few done on water fasting and the reason being is that people still believe water fasting is dangerous. However, the benefits associated with intermittent fasting would most definitely apply to people doing water fasting as well, and in fact potentially even more so.

For you to really achieve the most benefit from water fasting, you must follow a set number of rules and make sure that you follow my "preparing for the fast" and "breaking the fast" section as these are just as important.

The main benefit areas that will be covered in this book include the Brain, Immune System/Cancer and Fat Loss but additional benefits that water fasting has on your health will also be covered.

Chapter 4 – Benefits of Fasting – Brain Health

****

Fasting has been shown to be beneficial for the brain and central nervous system.

Let's take a look at our brains more a moment. They are miraculous organs which have an amazing capacity to maintain adequate sustenance during periods of scarcity. In today's society, with the excessive consumption of sugars and carbohydrates, we are constantly supplying our brains with steady streams of glucose by breaking down glycogen (a storage form of glucose primarily in the liver and muscles).

However, the problem with relying on glycogen stores is that it will only produce a short term availability of glucose. As the glycogen stores are depleted, the body will start to break down proteins through a process known as gluconeogenesis. This is a process that involves the breaking down of muscle tissue to provide glucose.

However, we have good news. The human physiology does offer another pathway to create energy for immediate use. Fasting is an exceptional way of pushing your body to go down this pathway instead. When food is no longer available (as is the case with a full water fast) the liver will begin to use body fat so as to create ketones. This generally takes about 48 hours for women and about 72 hours for men.

A particular ketone, known as beta hydroxybutyrate is a very efficient source of fuel for the brain and it allows people to function for extended periods of time during periods of food scarcity.

Apart from being an impressive fuel for the brain, studies have determined that beta hydroxybutyrate has other amazing benefits as well. Fasting, and therefore ketone production shifts the brains metabolism to enhance energy production and pave the way for better brain function and clarity, a decrease in depression and anxiety and even a reduction in insomnia.

Brain Benefit # 1 - Neuronal Autophagy

Autophagy, a process where the cells recycle waste materials, down regulate wasteful processes and repair themselves is increased during periods of fasting. In fact there have been studies showing that just eliminating an essential autophagy gene in rodents resulted in metabolic derangement in itself, as well as impaired neuronal development. Without the process of autophagy the brains are unable to develop properly nor function the way they should.

What is also interesting is that studies have shown that elevated levels of insulin actually reduce this process of autophagy.

Research (1) – "Short Term Fasting induces profound neuronal autophagy"

In this study they set out to determine if short term fasting leads to up regulation in neuronal autophagy and what they concluded was that fasting may in fact be a simple, safe and inexpensive means to promote the neuronal autophagy.

Brain Benefit #2 - Increases BDNF in the Brain

Fasting has been shown to increase BDNF levels in the brain. So, I can hear you asking right now – what is this BDNF thing you are talking about?

BDNF is Brain Derived Neurotrophic Factor, which is important for many different functions, including:

- Preventing the death of existing brain cells;
- Inducing the growth of new neurons; and
- Supporting cognitive function.

Low levels of BDNF are linked to Alzheimer's Disease and supplementary BDNF has been shown to prevent neuronal death, memory loss and cognitive impairment.

Research (2) – "Fasting and Exercise Differentially regulate BDNF mRNA expression in human skeletal muscle".

In this study they measured BDNF in human skeletal muscle following 3 intensities of exercise and a 48 hour fast. What they found was that there was no change in BDNF mRNA with exercise but fasting upregulated BDNF by 350%.

Brain Benefit #3 – Decreases Risk of Alzheimer's and Parkinson's Disease

Studies have found that fasting for a couple of days a week can help to protect yourself against the worst effects of Alzheimer's and Parkinson's Disease. Not only does the increase in BDNF, decrease in blood glucose and decrease in IGF all promote healthy brain function, but so does the increased production of ketones which are triggered by fasting.

Ketones have been shown to be beneficial in treating neurodegenerative diseases, in particular Alzheimer's and Epilepsy. In fact, the research study below has demonstrated how efficient ketones are for improvement in Alzheimer's disease.

Research (3) – "A new way to produce hyperketonemia: Use of ketone esters in a case of Alzheimer's Disease".

In this study, over a period of 20 months a potent ketogenic agent known as a ketone monoester was given by oral administration to a patient with Alzheimer's disease dementia. They found that the patient improved markedly in mood, self-care and cognitive and daily performance.

They also tracked plasma beta hydroxyl butyrate levels (indicators of ketone production) and what they found was noticeable improvements in conversation and interactions at higher levels in comparison to predose.

Brain Benefit #4 – Decreases Risk of Mental Decline and Memory Loss

Even when you do not suffer from neurodegenerative diseases, your mental ability naturally declines with age. However, it has been shown that intermittent fasting can improve mental functioning in ageing animals.

Research (4) – "Late-Onset Intermittent Fasting dietary restriction as a potential intervention to retard age-associated brain function impairment in male rats"

This study set out to determine what effect intermittent fasting later on in life would have on motor coordination and cognitive ability on ageing rats. What they found was this Intermittent Fasting decreased the Oxidative Stress within the brain as well as stopped age associated detrimental effects, such as cognitive and motor performance.

Brain Benefit #5 – Decreases Risk of Huntington's Disease

Although the number of studies done on fasting and Huntington's Disease in humans is minimal, there are studies out there which have been done on mice.

If reducing food intake has the same effect on humans as it does in the animal models, then it may be possible to delay the onset of Huntington's Disease and extend the lives of the patients.

There are three reasons why fasting is beneficial in regards to Huntington's Disease:

- Fasting seems to produce fewer degenerative nerve cells due to the fact that it is disposing of the cells that aren't required and healing the ones that it does.
- Fasting seems to elevate levels of HSP-70 (heat shock protein 70) which increases cellular resistance to stress. This protein seems to be less in those eating at will than those fasting.
- Fasting increases the level of BDNF, which stimulates the growth and survival of nerve cells. Therefore it may protect nerve cells from the adverse effects of the Huntington's gene.

These factors can be demonstrated in the animal research study below...

Research (5) – "Dietary restriction normalizes glucose metabolism and BDNF levels, slows disease progression and increases survival in huntington mutant mice".

In this study they took two groups of 8 week old mice (15 mice per group) who all had the huntingtons gene. One group was fed at will and the other group was maintained on an alternate day fasting regime where they fasted for 24 hours every other day.

In this study they found a number of different things happened:

- The onset of behavioral symptoms were significantly delayed in those mice that fasted.

- The survival time was extended in the fasted group. By 21 weeks of age all of those mice that were fed at will died while only 40% of those who fasted did.

- All the mice that had the Huntington's Gene exhibited weight loss but those that fasted lost less weight than those that didn't.

- Mice on the fasted regime exhibited highly significant improvements in motor performance.

- Expected brain atrophy was markedly less in those that fasted.

- Fasted Blood Glucose levels were lower on the mice that fasted.

- Levels of BDNF were increased 300-400% in mice that were fasted compared to the non-fasted mice.

- Levels of Heat Shock Protein was increased in the fasted mice.

Brain Benefit #6 – Decreases Risk of Stroke

Animal models of research have shown that fasting upregulated BDNF as well as a whole host of other neuroprotective proteins, reduced mortality and inflammation and increased cognitive health and function.

They also found that fasting decreased inflammatory cytokines, however this was modulated by age. In the studies they found that fasting was especially effective for those young mice and middle aged mice but not so effective for the elderly mice. Therefore, the effectiveness of fasting on stroke is dependent on age.

Research (6) – "Age and Energy Intake Interact To Modify Cell Stress Pathways and Stroke Outcome"

In this study they took 2 groups of mice of 3 different ages (3, 9 and 16 months) and put them on ad libitum (AL) or alternate day fasting (IF) for 4-5 months prior to the experimental stroke.

What they found was:
- Those young and middle aged mice on the fasting diet maintained significantly lower weights than those on the ad libitum diet.
- Blood Glucose concentrations were lower in those mice on the IF compared to AL regardless of age.
- Plasma Insulin levels were also significantly lower in all IF groups.
- The mice that were studied mimicked the most common type of human stroke "transient ischemia and reperfusion". After 1 hour of these mice having an ischemic attack, mortality rate during a 72 hour reperfusion was monitored. They found that mortality was affected by not only the diet, but also the age.
- Mortality was greater in the older mice (35%) compared to the younger mice (13%) and the middle aged mice (23%).
- Mortality was also greater in the AL group in comparison to all age groups of the IF group.
- The brain damage experienced was also less in the IF young and middle aged group than the AL group.
- In the elderly mice, IF had no significant effect on the brain damage.

Therefore this study showed that IF could be an effective treatment for the young and middle aged but maybe not so much for the elderly.

Brain Benefit #7 – Treating Brain Trauma

Research has shown that as fasting reduces oxidative stress, mitochondrial dysfunction and cognitive decline, it may be effective at helping with brain trauma.

Research (7) – "Fasting is Neuroprotective following traumatic brain injury"

In this study they investigated male rats to determine the neuroprotective effects of fasting after a traumatic brain injury. What they found was that fasting the animals for 24 hours resulted in a significant increase in tissue sparing, whereas 48 hours did not.

This 24 hour fast also decreased the biomarkers of oxidative stress and mitochondrial oxidative phosphorylation in the mitochondria.

The administration of ketones resulted in increased tissue sparing after moderate injury.

Brain Benefit #8 – Preventing and Treating Depression

Depression is a condition which is rising in occurrence every single day and it is one which is detracting from peoples quality of life. There are many reasons behind why somebody may be depressed and inflammation is one of them. Although it is unlikely that depression is an inflammatory disorder on its own, it is well known that many inflammatory conditions such as autoimmune diseases and heart disease can also have an element of depression wrapped into it.

One third of all people with major depression have been shown to have elevated levels of inflammation markers in the system, even in the absence of serious mental disorders. Studies have found that decreasing inflammatory cytokines can actually reduce the incidence of depression.

So in order to lower the rates of depression we must also lower the rates of inflammation in the body (which in turn will help people lose body fat, eliminate pain and overall have a better quality of life) and fasting has been shown to do just that.

Research (8) – "Interleukin 6, C-Reactive Protein and Biochemical Parameters during Prolonged Intermittent Fasting"

In this study they took 40 healthy participants of normal weight who fasted during Ramadan and another 28 healthy age and BMI matched volunteers who did not fast. They took blood samples one week prior to Ramadan, during the last week of Ramadan and 3 weeks after Ramadan had finished.

They measured IL-6, C-Reactive Protein, Homocysteine, Vitamin B12, Folate, Total Cholesterol, Triglycerides, HDL and LDL. The results of this study showed that no changes occurred in cholesterol levels BUT the triglyceride/HDL risk ratio was decreased during and after Ramadan in the fasting group but no changes in the non-fasting group.

On top of that the inflammatory markers IL-6, CRP and Homocysteine were significantly lower during Ramadan in the fasting group. This shows that fasting is effective at lowering inflammation and improving cardiovascular risk factors.

However, inflammation is not the only way that fasting can help Depression. Recent research has shown that low BDNF levels and Depression may actually be related. In fact it has been shown that one of the ways anti-depressants work is by increasing the level of BDNF in the body. Therefore it only seems plausible that increasing BDNF levels via fasting could help with depression.

Research (9) – "Decreased Serum Brain-Derived Neurotrophic Factor (BDNF) in major Depressed Patients."

In this study, 30 majorly depressed patients (15 male and 15 female) participated, as well as 30 healthy controls (15 male and 15 female). Serum BDNF was assayed with the use of the ELISA method and the severity of depression was evaluated.

What they found was that BDNF levels were significantly lower in patients than in controls. They also found that female patients were more depressed and released less BDNF than the men.

Brain Benefit #9 – Treating Epilepsy

For a while now Ketosis has been seen as a useful tool for the treatment of epilepsy. As fasting is effective at putting people into a ketotic state, it stands to reason that it is also useful for treating epilepsy. If undertaking a water fast it takes children only 1.5 days, women about 2 days and men about 3 days to enter ketosis.

Combining the Ketogenic Diet and Periodic Fasting together it provides an even greater chance of remission of epileptic seizures. It seems that the Ketogenic Diet and Fasting actually work in different ways when it comes to the nervous system and therefore they can be used in tandem.

Research (10) – "Seizures decrease rapidly after fasting – Preliminary Studies Of The Ketogenic Diet"

In this study the researchers set out to evaluate the changes in atonic or myoclonic seizures during the initiation of the ketogenic diet and after implementing fasting. In this study, children fasted for 36 hours so as to put them into a ketogenic state (one of the amazing benefits of fasting) and then gradually introduced the ketogenic diet over a period of 3 days. Parents were required to keep a baseline seizure frequency calendar to keep track of when the seizures occurred. They found that these seizures decreased in the children by more than 50% immediately.

Chapter 5 – Benefits of Fasting – Immune System/Cancer

Studies have shown that just by fasting for 3 days or longer, drinking only water and eating less than 200 calories per day you can seriously reset the components of the immune system. They found that fasting lowers white blood cells counts, therefore triggering the immune system to start producing new white blood cells.

Fasting forces your body to eliminate all of the immune cells that are not needed. Whilst fasting, an enzyme PKA and a hormone IGF-1 are reduced and so once you start eating again, these recycled cells will start to be replenished.

On top of that there are a number of other benefits that fasting provides for the immune system:

- Increases Macrophages;
- Decreases Antigen-Antibody Complexes;
- Increases Immunoglobulins;
- Increases Neutrophil Bactericidal Activity;
- Depresses Lymphocyte Blastogenesis;
- Heightens Monocyte Activity; and
- Enhances Natural Killer Cell Activity.

There are a number of specific immune related conditions that have been shown (both anecdotally and scientifically) to be helped or healed with fasting...

Immune Benefit #1 - Colds and Flu's

Do you remember a time when you were young and suffering from a fever and a host of other symptoms indicative of a cold or flu? Do you remember how little interest you had in food at that point? I know that when I am under the weather the last thing I want to do is eat.

Fasting is our body's natural way of fending off the cold or flu. It is an ancient remedy used for the healing of the common cold and although it is not well understood, most animals adhere to this healing principle.

If you feel like you are coming down with a cold, how about taking a day off of eating so as to give your body the chance to cleanse and heal itself a lot quicker.

Immune Benefit #2 - Autoimmune Disease

Conditions such as Rheumatoid Arthritis, Lupus, Crohns Disease, Psoriasis, Hashimotos Thyroiditis, Colitis and Asthma are all examples of Autoimmune Diseases.

As autoimmune disease is aggravated by leaky gut and fasting is effective at normalizing gut permeability, a water fast should be part of any treatment for autoimmune disease. By giving your digestive system a break from digesting food, it also allows time for your body to heal and seal the lining of your gut.

To read up on some case studies of people who have been able to reverse and/or treat their autoimmune diseases with water fasting, please read Chapter 7...

Immune Benefit #3 - Cancer

Fasting is a therapy that is continuing to be used for the treatment of cancer. Chemotherapy and other cancer treatments lower the functioning of the immune system and not only do these treatments kill the unhealthy cancer cells but they also kill off the healthy cells. By doing this they kill off the body's natural defenses against disease. By the end of the treatment cancer sufferers will have such a weakened immune system that they begin to take immune boosting supplements and medications instead.

Fasting forces your body to reboot the immune system and help to increase the production of white blood cells which have been destroyed in the cancer treatment. This will make it possible for the body to protect itself even after it has been flooded with chemo and radiation.

Fasting has also been found to be useful when it comes to minimizing the side effects associated with chemotherapy. If you would like to read some case studies on people who have used fasting alongside their cancer treatments so as to ease their symptoms and boost the immune system then please read Chapter 7...

Chapter 6 – Benefits of Fasting – Fat Loss
****

One of the greatest benefits associated with fasting is that of fat loss, and there are many ways that fasting achieves this:

Fat Loss Benefit #1 - Boosts Human Growth Hormone

The first way that fasting increases fat burning is through boosting Human Growth Hormone. It is well known that during a fast, Human Growth Hormone (HGH) – one of our premier fat burning hormones is increased.

Studies have shown that even a simple 24 hour fast increased growth hormone by 1300% in women and 2000% in men. This is great news for those wanting to lose that fat and build that muscle.

If you are still not 100% sure of what Human Growth Hormone is or what its benefits are, let me just go into it a little:

- Promotes the building of new muscle by increasing the synthesis of new protein tissues, such as in muscle recovery or repair.
- Produces more energy.
- Improves sexual performance.
- Builds stronger bones.
- Improves the quality and duration of heart and kidneys.
- Increases the breakdown of stored fats (triglycerides) and increases the use of this fat to create energy.
- Counteracts the action of insulin. Insulin moves sugar into the cells (i.e. stores fat) and Growth Hormone moves sugar out of the cells to be burned (i.e. fat burning).
- Human Growth Hormone reduces obesity because of its actions on two enzymes that control lipolysis (breakdown of stored triglycerides into free fatty acids) and lipogenesis (fat accumulation).

Research (11) – "Fasting enhances growth hormone secretion and amplifies the complex rhythms of growth hormone secretion in man"

> In this study they recruited 6 healthy males and collected their blood to test for 24 hour pulsatile patterns of growth hormone secretion, both during a control fed day and also during the first and fifth day of a 5 day fast.
>
> They found that the 5 day fast resulted in a significant increase in growth hormone pulse frequency, 24 hours growth hormone concentration and maximal pulse amplitude. They also found that fasting resulted in a decline in serum concentrations of somatomedin C (IGF-2) and glucose, as well as a rise in free fatty acids & acetoacetate.

Fat Loss Benefit #2 - Increases Lipolysis by Decreasing Insulin Levels

Lipolysis is the process of releasing stored triglycerides from the body (body fat) so that it may be burned for energy. However, when Insulin Levels are high, the process of Lipolysis is low, therefore making fat burning almost impossible. By lowering the insulin production through fasting, lipolysis is activated.

Fat Loss Benefit #3 - Improves Insulin Sensitivity

Insulin resistance has been linked to many conditions such as heart disease and diabetes, as well as a variety of cancers (prostate, breast and pancreatic). Fasting has been shown to improve insulin sensitivity and reduce insulin resistance.

Fat Loss Benefit #4 - Increases Catecholamine's and therefore activates Hormone Sensitive Lipase

Hormone Sensitive Lipase is present in the adipose tissues and is responsible for spurring the release of fat. The bodies Catecholamine's Adrenaline and Noradrenaline which are increased during fasting also increase this hormone sensitive lipase, therefore triggering the body to burn fat.

Fat Loss Benefit #5 - Burns More Calories

Short Term Fasting (between 12 hours and 72 hours) has been shown to increase your metabolism and adrenaline levels. This causes you to increase calorie burning during the period of the fast.

Fat Loss Benefit #6 - Trains your body to burn fat instead of sugar

As mentioned previously, once you shift your metabolism from burning sugars to burning fat (ketosis) you will be able to start tapping into stored body fat. By the end of the 24 hour fast your body has burnt more fat than you typically would in a normal day of eating.

The more days you fast the more keto-adapted you will become and therefore the more fat you will burn.

Chapter 7 – Benefits of Fasting – Other
****

On top of the beneficial effects of water fasting on the brain, immune system and obesity, there are also a host of other benefits:

- Ageing;

- Allergies;

- Cardiovascular Disease;

- Clearer Skin;

- Diabetes;

- Digestive Disorders;

- Drug Addictions;

- Exhaustion/Fatigue;

- Hypertension; and

- Sleep.

Chapter 8 – Case Studies – Autoimmune Disease

****

I thought it would be interesting for you to read up on case studies pertaining to people who have completed water fasts and achieved amazing results.

"Brief Case Reports of Medically Supervised Water Only Fasting Associated With Remissions of Autoimmune Disease"

Case #1 – Rheumatoid Arthritis

Initial Case
- 61 Year Old Man;
- Pain and Stiffness in all extremities, fatigue and headaches;
- Episodes of autoimmune hemorrhagic conjunctivitis;
- Was on 100mg cyclosporine and 5mg prednisone daily.
- Began fasting 1 month after stopping medications.
- Initial weight was 71.8kg and Blood pressure was 110/60.

Results
- Within 2 days of fasting, joint symptoms started to subside.
- After a week of fasting, he had no pain and mobility was returned.
- By the 8th day there was a brief recurrence of conjunctivitis.
- He fasted for a total of 17 days.
- After the fast he had no residual symptoms.
- His weight was 63.4kg and blood pressure was 90/60.

Case #2 – Mixed Connective Tissue Disease

Initial Case
- 38 year old woman.
- Severe joint paints, facial edema, weakness, fatigue, chills, photosensitivity.
- Taking hydroxychloroquine, tramadol, levothyroxine, cetirizine, and prednisone.
- Before the fast, she was taken off of all medications except thyroid meds which were reduced during the fast and raised to normal dose after the fast.
- Weight was 68.1kg and blood pressure was 115/80.

Results
- At the onset of the fast she had increased hip pain and discomfort as well as muscle weakness.
- Overall ill feeling during the first week of fasting.
- By the 10th day she felt better and after 21 days she had no further complaints.
- Weight dropped to 58.8kg and blood pressure was 80/60.
- At follow up she remained free of medication with minimal symptoms.

Case #3 – Fibromyalgia

Initial Case
- 46 year old woman.
- History of poor sleep and pain, especially in the right arm, back and neck and both legs.
- Could not sustain any activity for more than an hour.
- Medications included nefazodone, nortriptryline, propoxyphene, ibuprofen and levothyroxine.
- Weight was 67.2kg and blood pressure was 120/80.

Results
- Fast lasted 24 days, after which she was symptom free.
- At discharge her weight was 57.9kg and blood pressure was 115/85.
- At the follow up visit 1 month later she was symptom free.

Case #4 – Systemic Lupus Erythematosus

Initial Case
- 45 year old woman.
- Joint pain, chest pain and skin rash.
- Medications included 25mg of prednisone and 5mg of hydroxychloroquine daily.
- Was weaned off of medications 2 months prior to the fast and was medication free 2 weeks prior.
- Her initial weight was 58.8kg and blood pressure was 120/75.

Results
- During the first 3 days she experienced mild discomfort, poor sleep and nausea.
- By the fourth day, she was feeling significantly better with no complaints and no joint pain.
- Fast was broken on 7th day because of increased weakness and mild tachycardia.
- Weight was 55kg and blood pressure 110/80.
- Prolonged use of prednisone possibly caused adrenal exhaustion.
- She was symptom free for a year when her symptoms began to recur.
- Underwent a second 7 day fast and now has no symptoms.

Case #5 – Rheumatoid Arthritis

Initial Case
- 40 year old woman.
- Pain in all joints, especially the knees.
- Weight at the start was 71.8kg and blood pressure 125/100.

Results
- In the first few days of the fast there was increased pain in the spine, shoulders and neck.
- Pain decreased as the fast continued and by day 10 there was no further joint pain.
- Fasted for 12 days.
- Weight went down to 65kg and blood pressure 110/70.
- Symptoms have not recurred.

Case #6 – Rheumatoid Arthritis

Initial Case
- 46 year old woman.
- Pain in the fingers, wrists, shoulders and knees.
- Medications include irbesartan, amlodipine, celecoxib, rofecoxib.
- Weight was 106.6kg and blood pressure 170/80.

Results
- Weaned off all medications and put on a dietary regime for 8 weeks prior to the fast. She lost 9.1kg during this time.
- At the start of the fast, her weight was 94.5kg and blood pressure without medications was 130/78.
- Within 4 days of the fast her joint pain decreased.
- Her symptoms continued to decrease throughout the fast.
- She fasted for 24 days and had no residual symptoms.
- Her weight dropped to 84.3kg and blood pressure normalized to 110/80.
- Still in remission.

So, as you can see by all of these case studies, water fasting has been shown to be incredibly beneficial when it comes to autoimmune disease. And don't worry, if you have an autoimmune disease that is not listed here it is important to understand that it really doesn't matter. Autoimmune Disease is the same illness but with different names depending on the part of the body your immune system is attacking.

Even though Hashimoto's Thyroiditis or Multiple Sclerosis are not listed here does not mean water fasting does not work for people suffering from these conditions. I know that it helps my Hashimoto's. Does it help your autoimmune condition? Please let me know by emailing jen@asknaturopathjen.com and I will try to start a collection of testimonials to put in the book.

Chapter 9 – Case Studies – Cancer
****

Case #1 – Breast Cancer

Initial Case
- 51 year old Caucasian woman with Stage 2A Breast Cancer.
- Was receiving adjuvant chemotherapy consisting of docetaxel and cyclophosphamide.
- Fasted prior to her first chemotherapy administration.
- Fasting regimen consisted of a water fast for 140 hours (5.8 days) prior to chemotherapy and 40 hours (1.6 days) after chemotherapy and only consumed water and vitamins.

Results
- She completed this fast with little inconvenience and lost 7 pounds which were put back on by end of treatment.
- After the first fasting-chemo cycle she experienced mild fatigue, dry mouth and hiccups but was still able to carry out daily activities.
- However in the second and third treatment she received chemotherapy as well as a regular diet and complained of moderate to severe fatigue, weakness, nausea, abdominal cramps and diarrhea. She was not able to maintain a normal schedule.
- In the fourth cycle she opted to fast again but this time 120 hours prior to the chemotherapy and 24 hours after chemotherapy. Side effects were lower here, despite the expected cumulative toxicity from previous cycles.
- They found total white blood cell and absolute neutrophil counts were slightly better when chemo was preceded by fasting. Also platelets dropped by 7-19% during cycles 2 and 3 but not 1 and 4. After the fourth cycle combined with the 144 hour fast her white blood cells, neutrophils and platelets reached their highest levels since chemo started 80 days previously.

Case #2 – Esophageal Adenocarcinomametastasic in Adrenal Glands

Initial Case
- 68 year old Caucasian male.
- 5-fluorouracil and cisplatin concurrent with radiation for first two cycles.
- During the first two cycles the patient experienced severe weakness, fatigue, mucositis, vomiting and grade 2-3 peripheral neuropathy.
- During the third cycle 5-FU was discontinued due to severe nausea and refractory vomiting and in spite of the aggressive radiation and chemo his disease progressed with new metastases to right adrenal gland, lung nodules, left sacrum and coracoid process.
- During fourth cycle he started taking carboplatin in combination with TAX and 5-FU. However, he incorporated a 72 hour fast prior to chemo and a 51 hour fast afterwards.

Results
- Patient lost 7 pounds of which 4 were regained after resuming the diet.
- Side effects were less severe than when food was consumed.
- Prior to 5th cycle he opted to fast again. However, instead of receiving the 5-FU infusion for 96 hours, it was administered for 48 hours, alongside a 48 hour water fast and 56 hour fast after the chemotherapy was administered.
- Side effects were once again less severe than when eating.
- He proceeded to fast throughout cycles 6,7,8 with minimal side effects except for mild diarrhea and abdominal cramps.
- Unfortunately the patient's disease progressed and died in February 2009. However, at least it meant that he suffered with less side effects than he would have if he hadn't of fasted so it gave him better quality of life.

You can find more Cancer Case Studies at http://www.ncbi.nlm.nih.gov/pmc/articles/PMC2815756/

Chapter 10 – Deciding If A Fast Is Right For You

****

Although I believe that a fast is beneficial for most people, it is not always the right time and there are certain people that should not be doing a fast.

But before I go into the people that shouldn't be doing a water fast, how about I go into the people who I believe should be doing one.

Who Should Fast...?

Are you suffering from an Autoimmune Condition that leaves you in chronic pain every day?

If so, fasting has been shown to alleviate pains associated with autoimmune disease as well as modulate the immune system and in some cases even reverse autoimmune disease (See Chapter 4).

Are you struggling to lose the fat and just need a little kick start?

Water fasts have an innate ability to push you into ketosis quite quickly, therefore helping to train your body to burn fat a lot quicker.

Are you run down and tired every day and want to feel more energized?

By allowing your body to move away from focusing all of its attention on digestion, it can focus more attention on the energy systems within the body and therefore help you feel more energized and on the ball.

Are you so emotionally connected to food that you don't even know how you are going to go the next hour without it?

If so, it is likely you have a food addiction. What is the number one thing you need to do to get over an addiction of any type? That's right – abstinence.

If you are addicted to carbohydrates, you abstain from them, if you are addicted to drugs, you abstain from them and the same applies to food.

By abstaining from eating for a period of time not only will your hunger disappear within the first few days of the fast (therefore minimizing you thinking about it) but you will also learn to appreciate other things around you other than food.

Are you going through cancer treatment and suffering extreme side effects?

As you can see by Chapter 4, there are many people who have indicated that fasting alongside conventional therapies have really helped them settle down the uncomfortable side effects AND improve the outcome.

OR

Are you just wanting to improve your overall health and longevity?

These are just some of the examples of who would want to fast. Maybe you want to fast to improve your mental clarity and creativity or maybe it is to really get in touch with your spiritual side.

However, no matter what the reason is, it is important that you do it safely and if you are doing it for longer than 5 days I would recommend you speak to a qualified practitioner when doing it.

Also make sure that you follow the directions I give in the "Preparing for a Fast", "Completing the Fast" and "Breaking the Fast" section as I give tips on the safest and most beneficial way of completing a water fast. Please note that Water Fasting is incredibly safe and beneficial if done properly.

Situations When Fasting May Be Contraindicated

Who Should Not Fast

If you have liver or kidney disease or are frail, malnourished, anemic or adrenally exhausted then you should not do a fast at this point in time. It is important to get those issues in check first.

Who Should Fast with Supervision

If you have a weakened immune system, severely high blood pressure, medication dependent diabetes or a weak circulation, you should only do a fast under the supervision of your doctor.

When Sleep Deprived/Stressed

If you are sleep deprived or stressed then it is advisable to get a handle on your sleep and stress prior to starting the fast but if not ensure that during the fast you incorporate some meditation, prayer, self-hypnosis, relaxation, light walking and play so as to lower those stress levels and ensure you are getting good quality sleep.

Initially fasting can be seen as a stress on the system so adding more on top of your current stress level can aggravate things. It is incredibly important to remain as stress free as possible during that time.

Children

Although the need for a child to fast is relatively rare they are able to do so safely as long as they are monitored sufficiently. For infants, 2-3 days is fine and for children 1-2 weeks is a good duration. I know that my daughter fasts on the odd occasion with me when she is not feeling well and she feels more energized and alive when she does so.

Monitor your child when they are doing it and if they start to feel dizzy and lightheaded then give them a little salt and if they still don't feel well then break that fast ASAP. Your child will tell you when they don't feel well. It is really important though that you make sure you have them do the fast as it is mentioned in this book and remember if ever you are worried about anything then always see your practitioner.

Pregnancy

If you are pregnant then it has been shown to be perfectly fine, and possibly even beneficial to fast as long as you are not diabetic. Make sure that if you do choose to fast during this time that you are doing so under the supervision of your medical practitioner and that you do not fast for any longer than 5 days at a time.

Chapter 11 – Preparing For A Water Fast

Step #1 – Work out The Details

How long are you going to do the fast for? Are you going to start off with a short fast and then work up to a longer fast? If this is your first time doing a water fast I would recommend you start off with maybe a 1 or 2 day fast and then work your way up to a 10 day fast.

However, it is also possible to jump straight in to a 10 day fast once you have tackled the rest of the "preparing for the fast" steps.

When are you going to begin the fast?

To be fully prepared for the fast and have less side effects, you need to allow yourself at least 2 weeks prior to starting the water fast to ease into it. If you do not, you may find that your "healing crisis" may be a lot worse.

What Issues are you hoping to fix with the fast?

Write down a long list of what you are hoping to achieve with the fast. Do you have joint pains that you are wanting to eliminate, do you have skin issues, what about an autoimmune condition you are looking at reversing. Are you doing it just to kick start that fat loss and lose a few kg. Whatever your reasons are, write them down in a journal so you can keep tabs on how everything is going as the fast continues.

Step #2 – Work out your Schedule

Now that you have decided when you are going to do the fast, make sure that you have absolutely nothing on socially during that period of time. There is nothing worse than having to go out to dinner with friends and do nothing but drink water. The time spent during your water fast should be relaxing time with minimal commitments.

Of course, I don't expect you to give up work, especially if you are doing a 10 day fast but if you are only going to start off with a 2 day fast, then doing it on the weekend is a great idea.

Step #3 – Prepare Your Mindset

This may sound hair fairy but there are going to be some changes that happen, especially in the first few days. If you are not prepared mentally for these changes you may give up on the fast too soon thinking that you are harming your body or that you are not receiving the benefits you should be.

To prepare your mindset there are a few things I recommend:

Accept that there are going to be some unwanted effects in the first few days.

Healing Crisis

While your body is switching from being a sugar burner to a fat burner you may experience detox symptoms (also known as a healing crisis). Some of these symptoms include headache, nausea, vomiting, diarrhea and skin eruptions. These are all signs that you are detoxing the harmful substances from your system to make way for regeneration and repair.

To minimize these effects it is a good idea to become ketogenic prior to the fast.

Dizziness

Sometimes you may also experience light headedness and dizziness caused from low blood pressure. Fasting is known to lower your blood pressure which is great if you have hypertension BUT if you have normal or low blood pressure this can become an issue.

If you find that you get dizzy when you get up too quickly then it is an idea to make sure you get up very slowly and pause between postures to give your body the chance to adjust to the changes in gravity. At the first sign of dizziness put your head between your knees so that your head is lower than your heart.

Back Pain

If you are doing a longer fast you may find that you start to experience some back pain. This is normal and will pass and is actually because of overworked kidneys. Your kidneys have been working hard at eliminating all of the toxins from your body. Make sure that you are drinking plenty of fluids and use some hot baths or hot water bottles to provide relief.

Less Sleep Requirement

Although you may want to sleep more (to make the time pass) you may find that you actually require less sleep. It is important that you rest plenty but you may find that sleep is not as necessary during this period as your body is already rested.

Low Grade Aches and Pains

As you proceed through your fast you may notice that the organ or body part which is diseased will begin to ache. However as you go on with the fast these aches will usually lessen until they are not there anymore. Use hot water bottles, hot baths and possibly some magnesium oil to help with these aches and pains.

Intense Hunger

During the first 2-3 days of the fast you are going to experience hunger and cravings as your body is still surviving on glucose. However, once it realizes that there is no glucose there and all of the glycogen has been used up it will start to shift to a fat burning state where it will begin to burn ketones and your hunger will begin to disappear.

Glucose is no longer needed.

Get yourself a journal

It is very common during a fast that you will begin to unravel emotions that you didn't even know existed. You may start to cry, you may begin to feel anxious and you may even feel emotional swings which are very concerning. However, it is important to understand that this is normal.

When you fast you are not only detoxing your body but also detoxing your mind. There could be a physical aspect involved where the drugs and pharmaceuticals you have been taking previously are now being released from the fat cells or it could be mental where you are getting in touch with your spiritual and emotional side now that food is not in the way. Whatever it is, just go with it, allow those feelings to pass and it will get better, with you most likely feeling more alive and refreshed at the end of it.

These strong emotional swings will vary from person to person and can also vary in intensity. In some people it may not happen at all.

However, if the emotions become too strong be prepared to end the fast.

I like to get myself a journal to record my whole fasting experience so that I can monitor these feelings and possibly resolve some long hidden issues. Review these feelings at the end of the fast and you may even get a message out of it.

Prepare yourself to meditate

When you are fasting you may find that you are able to get into a meditative state a lot quicker and you will experience a level of clarity and awareness that you have never experienced before. When your body is no longer having to focus on digestion, it is able to experience the higher meditative states a lot easier.

If you are not yet meditating, during the fast is the ideal time to start.

Not only will you find it easier to clear the mind and focus on the one act of meditation, but you will also have the extra time in the day to do it.

Step #4 - Prepare Your Nutrition

Reduce all of your habitual and addictive substances 1-2 weeks prior to the fast

If you are still smoking, drinking or consuming stimulants such as caffeine and soft drinks then a couple of weeks prior to doing the water fast you should reduce and if possible eliminate those substances. The more that you reduce the junk foods and garbage that you put in your body, the easier it is going to be for your body to cleanse during the fast.

By reducing or possibly eliminating these addictive substances prior to the fast you will not experience the withdrawal symptoms from these products as well as the symptoms associated with the fast itself.

Follow a Keto Plan 1-2 weeks prior to the fast

This makes sense doesn't it? With the fast we are trying to get our body to burn as much fat as possible and start using ketones as quickly as possible so that we may not experience the hunger associated with it.

Therefore, it is recommended that you severely eliminate the sugars and starches for a couple of weeks prior so that your body is already burning ketones when you begin the fast. This will negate any of the sugar withdrawal effects that occur when your body is going from a sugar burner to a fat burner as it is already burning fat. It will also eliminate the hunger and will make the fast a lot easier.

It can take some people up to 2 weeks to become fat adapted on the ketogenic diet but with others it can take just a few days. You can check with a ketone meter if you are not unsure whether you are fat adapted yet.

If you are not yet sure how to begin a ketogenic diet you can get my books "Understanding Keto" (Beginners Guide to the Ketogenic Diet) or "Keto Blocks" (40 Reasons why you may be plateauing on the Ketogenic Diet).

Follow A Real Food Soup Plan a couple of days before the Water Fast

It is very important that a couple of days prior to you starting the fast that your digestive system is prepared. This means that you need to eliminate the poor quality foods a couple of days prior to the fast (I assume you won't have too many of them as you are on keto already).

Many people recommend juice fasts prior to a water fast because of its ease on digestion. While I do recommend green vegetable juices I do not recommend fruit juices due to the fact that it is extremely high in sugar and will kick you out of ketosis almost immediately.

Instead I recommend low carb vegetable soups with added coconut milk or coconut cream (good for digestion) and maybe 1 or 2 green juices a day. I know this is restrictive but it will make the symptoms associated with the fast a lot better.

Step #5 – Prepare The Environment

Pre Cook Your Families Meals

If you are married and/or have children it is a good idea that prior to the fast you prepare some meals and freeze them. The last thing you are going to want to do is look at food – at least in the first few days of the fast.

If you are doing a longer fast you may find that after a few days you don't care for food anyway and so it is fine. But definitely for the first few days have the dinners pre-cooked so that your significant other or your children can get them out and heat them up.

From personal experience, I prefer not to watch them when they are eating and I am doing a water fast. Therefore at dinner time I leave them to their own devices, go and run myself a bath with my bottle of water and listen to a meditation track.

Teach your kids to make their own Breakfast and Lunch

If you have children that are older it is a good idea to ask them to prepare breakfast for themselves. With my children they are old enough that they can cook their own eggs, prepare their own fruit and yogurt and even heat up some soup.

On the odd occasion they may also help themselves to some gluten free cereal. For lunches I always make sure there are soups available and my kids know how to make up a salad. After all, it is only for a few days. If it is the weekend, maybe you can ask your spouse to prepare those two meals for them for those couple of days.

This will make it easier than once again having to look at food when you are hungry.

Create a Sleep Sanctuary

As mentioned previously, when fasting you often require less sleep. This does not mean you shouldn't attempt to get the best quality sleep you can. Create a space in your room that is relaxing and a haven for you. The bedroom should only ever be used for two things, and that is sleep and sex.

So make sure that it is warm and inviting and a place that you would like to go to at night.

It is important during this time of fasting that you optimize the sleep you are getting and although you may not require as many hours, you are going to need to get into the Non Rem sleep as much as possible which is the reparative and healing sleep.

If you are interested in learning more about sleep, please sign up for my main mailing list at http://www.lowcarbketoliving.com/freelist and you will be informed about when my new sleep course and webinars are coming up.

Step #6 – See Your Practitioner

Water fasting is extremely safe if done properly but there are some people who should definitely seek help from their practitioner first (please see Chapter #9). If you fit into this category, please make sure that you are monitored by a practitioner.

It is completely safe to do a water fast up to 3 days without the need to see a practitioner. However if you are intending on a longer fast it may be wise to consult with a practitioner (GP, Naturopath etc.) and have them monitor you.

I always recommend that you get a full blood panel consisting of:

- Inflammatory Markers (HS-CRP, Homocysteine);
- Cholesterol (HDL, Triglycerides);
- Thyroid Hormones (TSH, T3, T4, Reverse T3);
- Immune Health (Full Blood Count); and
- Auto Antibodies (Autoimmunity).

You can then have your bloods re-collected after the fast and compare the numbers.

If you are taking medications it is important to speak to your doctor about whether it is OK to take them during a fast or not. Many medications are able to be taken on an empty stomach and I suspect these would be fine but as I am not a medical doctor I cannot say for sure so speak to your GP and see what they recommend.

Step #7 – Prepare Your Body

There are a couple of things you should do to prepare your body:

Weigh yourself and take some measurements as it will be interesting to see the changes that have been made over the course of the fast.

About 12 hours prior to starting the plan, it is an idea to take a laxative so that you can eliminate any built up waste products in your system.

Chapter 12 – Completing The Water Fast

Now that you have prepared for the fast and you are sure today is the day, then let's get started.

Completing a water fast is really pretty simple in principle. It involves consuming water and nothing else for the period that you have decided on.

Step #8 – Drink the Right Water

Type of Water

You need to find the best quality water you can possibly find. It is important to drink pure water during this process so that your body has the ability to cleanse it as efficiently as possible.

Bottled Water

Bottled water may be OK if you are sure it is not just bottled tap water. I have a product here called "Pureau" which I have researched and it is guaranteed to be 100% free of all bacteria, chlorine, fluoride, salt and other impurities. This is the water I use when I am water fasting. Of course it does cost a bit but it is well worth it.

Filtered Water

This is a step above tap water, as long as it is significantly purer than that coming out of the tap. Most carbon filters eliminate a majority of the chlorine and bacteria so that is fine.

Tap Water

If you really do not have access to anything other than tap water then use that. The water fast is still going to provide remarkable benefits anyway.

Distilled Water

Although distilled water is great at binding to toxins and eliminating them from the body, they are also efficient at removing all electrolytes from the water, therefore making it dangerous for long term fasts.

Without sufficient electrolytes you will suffer from high blood pressure and heartbeat irregularities. It may be worthwhile drinking distilled water only for the first day or two to help eliminate the toxins and then switch across to one of the other types of water. Do not use distilled water for the entire fast as it could be dangerous.

Quantity of Water

Just because all that you are consuming is water does not mean that you should go and drink 4 liters of it a day. In fact there is a condition known as hyponatremia which can occur in people that consume too much water at any given time.

This condition also known as water intoxication is a potentially fatal disturbance in the brain that will result when the electrolytes in the body are pushed outside the safe limits by consuming too much water.

When water is over consumed in a specific amount of time it can actually be considered a poison. As the kidneys of a healthy person is really only able to excrete a maximum of 1 liter of water per hour I would not exceed that amount. In fact I would say that any more than a glass an hour is not necessary.

When water fasting it is not necessary to drink a particular amount of water. I would suggest up to 8 glasses a day is sufficient but if you are still thirsty you could get away with a little more. Just drink as much water as is comfortable with you. If you are running to the toilet every 5 minute, cut back a little bit.

Step #9 – Integrate Activity

Just because you are fasting does not mean you need to become a hermit. In fact, when I am water fasting I try to walk as much as I possibly can. I do not recommend that you start a P90x or a Turbo fire when water fasting as you will generally have a greater level of weakness (at least for the first week or so) but I definitely recommend going out into the fresh air and going on some nice long walks.

When I am fasting I will often walk for 2 or 3 hours a day. It distracts my mind from thinking about food, it will help to burn those extra calories and as I am out in nature I am breathing in some great quality air.

I am always exercising in places where there are a lot of trees and beautiful surroundings so that I can meditate while doing so. If you are in the city this may be a little more difficult, but still getting outside and incorporating some activity can make a huge difference on how you feel, how you sleep and how beneficial your fast is for you.

Step #10 – Get Productive – Now....

Fasting brings about a sense of calmness and creativity that is not achieved when you are consuming food. Use this time of creativity during the fast to tackle the biggest business goal you have. If you are writing a book then this is the time to do it. If you are finishing a piece of art, then fasting whilst doing so can really help. No matter what it is, give it a go. In fact, many artists deliberately fast during times when they are wanting to be the most creative.

Also, as you will most likely be sleeping less, that leaves more time for you to achieve those goals you have set for yourself.

Step #11 – Keep Yourself Busy

One of the most important things I have discovered through water fasting is that at least for the first few days you need to keep yourself really busy. Spring Clean the house, Get out in the garden or Organize that filing system. No matter what it is, keeping yourself occupied doing other things will keep your mind off of the food.

Step #12 – Relax and Meditate

As I mentioned previously it is a great time to really learn how to meditate. You can do this using the meditation CD's that are sent to you by signing up for my list or else use your own. For more information on this, you can check out the section on Meditation in the "Preparation" section.

Chapter 13 – Exiting The Water Fast

It is very important that when you have finished your fast you do not overburden your digestive system by going straight out and eating solid foods.

You must take it slow and remember that during the fast you would have created this new relationship with how you approach food.

Therefore, you don't want to go straight out and start your old binge eating habits again.

While you have been fasting you need to remember that the digestive enzymes that were once active have not been required and therefore have ceased to be produced. Therefore, introducing the foods slowly is of utmost importance.

On top of that, the lining of the stomach may have reduced function as it hasn't needed to be used for a while and therefore you need to be gentle with it when you are reintroducing the foods. Avoid foods that are irritating to the stomach such as coffee and spicy foods.

I just wanted to point out that now that you have received all of the amazing fat burning benefits of the ketogenic diet, you may decide that you do not want to go back to being a sugar burner and may decide to continue on with the ketogenic diet. If so then you can check out either of my books "Understanding Keto" or "Keto Blocks" which will explain a lot more.

Otherwise, if you do not need to be as restrictive you can instead lean more towards paleo and reintroduce some fruits and starchy vegetables into the mix.

No matter which plan you choose, please don't reintroduce junk foods into your plan. You have spent all this time and energy detoxing your body and bringing yourself back to health that you don't want to backtrack.

Avoid gluten at all costs and eliminate any other foods you may be intolerant to, such as dairy or eggs. In many cases, the water fast may have rectified some of those intolerances anyway.

Overeating when breaking a fast is even worse than overeating at any other time and therefore you should really follow this step when breaking your fast...

Step #13 – Integrate Foods Slowly

DAY ONE - Break your fast with only vegetable juices and bone broths. This gives your stomach and your enzymes the ability to come back to normal.

DAY TWO - Next you can move on to cooked vegetables and vegetable soups.

DAY THREE – Raw Vegetables.

DAY FOUR + - Normal Eating.

Chapter 14 – Summary Of The 13 Steps To A Successful Water Fast

****

PREPARATION

1. Work out the Details
2. Work out Your Schedule
3. Prepare Your Mindset
4. Prepare Your Nutrition
5. Prepare Your Environment
6. See Your Practitioner
7. Prepare Your Body

COMPLETE THE FAST

8. Drink the Right Water
9. Maintain Activity
10. Become Productive, Now…
11. Keep Busy…
12. Relax and De-stress

BREAKING THE FAST

13. Integrate Foods Slowly

Chapter 15 – Common Fasting Questions Answered

****

Q1. Will my metabolism slow down if I don't eat?

This is one of the greatest myths out there and is still being promoted by many fitness experts and personal trainers.

For years I heard that to lose weight you need to eat 6 times a day so that you can keep the fires burning. However, eating 3 meals a day as opposed to 6 meals has absolutely no effect on fat loss as long as the number of calories are the same. Metabolic rate is determined by the amount of calories you consume in each meal not the frequency of those meals.

To demonstrate that please refer to the research study below:

Research (12) – "Increased Meal Frequency Does Not Promote Greater Weight Loss in Subjects Who Were Prescribed an 8 Week Equi-Energetic Energy Restricted Diet"

In this study they set out to determine if there was in fact an inverse relationship between meal frequency and adiposity. They wanted to determine whether a higher meal frequency (3 meals and 3 snacks) could lead to a greater weight loss than low meal frequencies (3 meals).

They split the subjects into 2 separate groups with exactly the same amount of calories per day, for a period of 8 weeks.

What they found was that there was a similar decrease in body weight, fat mass and BMI but there were no significant differences between the low meal frequency and high meal frequency group, in regards to adiposity.

Q2. Will my body think it is starving if I fast?

No, your body will not think that it is starving if you undertake a water fast. So that I can demonstrate why, let me go into how fasting and starvation differ.

When we don't consume food, such as in fasting, the body will manage to cleanse itself of everything except those tissues which are vital.

Starvation will only occur if the body is forced to use these vital tissues to survive.

When we think of how much extra fat we have on our body I would think that we would be able to survive for an extended period of time without our body needing to feed on our tissues. Researchers have stated that as humans adapt very well to a lack of food, the average person would actually be able to survive for up to 75 days without it.

In fact, the heavier you are, the longer you should realistically be able to survive without food.

This is not to say however that I recommend water fasting for 75 days.

A fast of 10 – 21 days is sufficient time to be able to achieve the benefits associated with water fasting.

So, when is it that you will enter starvation mode? That would be when you no longer have the fat to be used for energy. But even the slimmest of people could probably survive for at least the 10 day period and possibly even longer. Every pound of fat that we carry on our body is worth 3500 calories so 1 pound of extra fat would be enough for us to handle physical labor for an entire day without consuming anything else.

The research study below shows how metabolism actually increases in a short term fast all the way up to 72 hours. This might be a good reason to do regular 2-3 day water fasts.

Research (13) – "The Cardiovascular, Metabolic and Hormonal Changes Accompanying Acute starvation in men and women"

In this study they took 29 healthy subjects (17 women and 12 men) and they tested the effect of fasting for 12, 36 and 72 hours. Measurements that were made during this time were cardiovascular variables, metabolic rate, respiratory exchange ratio, plasma metabolites, insulin, thyroid hormones and catecholamines.

During the 12-72 hour period they found:
1. No significant changes in blood pressure;
2. Heart rate increased at 36 hours and remained elevated after 72 hours.
3. Metabolic Rate was significantly increased after 36 hours of starvation but after 72 hours it was not significantly different than at 12 hours.
4. Plasma insulin and T3 fell during the fasting period and adrenalin and noradrenalin increased after the 72 hours.

Q3. Will fasting cause muscle loss?

Although many believe that fasting will cause you to lose muscle due to the lack of protein, I am here to tell you that once you become fat adapted, most of your energy demands will be met by stored fat and ketones and therefore protein will not be required to spare muscle. Fat adaptation and fasting are actually protein sparing.

However, if you are a sugar burner this is a completely different story. In this case your body is unable to tap into the fat stores as efficiently and therefore will require protein as their glucose source in the case of fasting. Remember however that within the first 2 days you will switch across to becoming a fat burner and therefore you will get the protein sparing effects anyway.

Now if you are concerned about muscle loss during fasting it is interesting to know that Dr Joel Furhman who is a respected MD and has done extensive research on fasting and nutrition states that muscle loss decreases to 0.2kg per day once you have reached full ketosis.

Another MD known as Peter Sultana predicts that you could probably go up to 40 days before you start to really catabolize muscle for fuel.

Once you have reached 80% of your ideal body weight, you will now enter starvation mode.

Therefore, there is really no need to be overly concerned about losing muscle during a water fast.

Q4. How does fasting affect your cortisol levels?

Yes, water fasting can increase your level of cortisol if it is extended (as in over 3 days) but this can be reduced by taking some branched chain amino acids during the fast. It is very important that you do not begin to undertake a water fast (or any fast for that matter) when you are sleep deprived, overly stressed or in a busy period of your life.

You need to minimize as many external stressors as you can during this period and implement relaxation strategies such as meditation and yoga to help balance the cortisol out. Remember that once the fasting period has stopped, so will the cortisol spikes.

Q5. Will I put the weight back on once I go off the fast?

The quick answer to this question is "it depends". If you go back to eating the foods that you ate prior to the fast then yes you will put the weight back on. I find that if after you complete the fast you continue to eat ketogenic then the amount of weight you put on will be minimal.

However, if you choose to eat more carbohydrates then you are going to put more weight on. Eating the carbohydrates will refill your glycogen, increase your insulin and decrease fat burning (therefore increase the amount of weight gain).

Q6. Doesn't the brain require glucose to function?

As mentioned previously, if you are fat adapted then your brain is perfectly capable of using fatty acids and ketones for fuel and therefore does not require the glucose to function.

Within the first couple of days of being on a water fast you will become keto adapted and your brain will begin to be able to function perfectly.

Note however that during those first couple of days you may feel lightheaded, dizzy and hungry due to hypoglycemia but that will rectify itself once you become keto adapted. Just try to make sure that during those first few days you relax as much as you can.

Q7. Won't I become nutrient deficient if I fast?

Actually, No you won't become nutrient deficient if you fast. In fact, there have been many cases of people whose nutrient deficiencies have actually improved after doing a water fast.

As we break down fat during the fast, tiny amounts of muscle (0.2kg per day), as well as a whole host of other tumors, cysts and lipomas that we don't require in our body are also broken down.

During this process, nutrients will be released in the bloodstream and become available for the body to reuse.

If you are doing a shorter fast it is likely you still have enough nutrients floating around in your bloodstream and if you are doing a longer fast you will receive these nutrients through the process described above.

Our body usually has plenty of minerals floating around at any one time and when our body is fasting, cleansing and healing, it becomes much more efficient at utilizing them.

Therefore, you will often see people who are deficient in something such as B12 or Iron become higher in that vitamin/mineral than they were previously.

Q8. Should I take supplements during my fast?

Although it is not necessary to take supplements when you are fasting it is up to the individual. It is not going to hamper your fast as long as you are taking supplements that are able to be absorbed on an empty stomach.

There are certain supplements, like Vitamin D, Vitamin K, Vitamin A and Vitamin E (fat soluble vitamins) that should be taken with food and therefore it would not be worthwhile taking them when fasting.

Supplements in themselves are not going to halt the fast as long as they are not supplements that trigger gluconeogenesis in the body (such as glutamine).

During a fast I myself supplement with MSM, Lysine (ketogenic amino acid), Vitamin C, Magnesium and Vitamin B.

Q9. Is fasting really necessary. Doesn't the body detox itself?

Yes, when we are healthy our body has the ability to detoxify itself.

However, due to sub-optimal lifestyle habits, as well as poor food choices, our body becomes less and less able to eliminate these cellular wastes on an ongoing basis.

Because of this, the cells become surrounded by these wastes and negatively impact the ability of the cells to do their job correctly.

However, the health issues we experience are not just caused from the poor food choices and the inability for our body to detoxify properly, but it is because of the massive amounts of toxins in our environment.

Not only are we surrounded by radiation and pollution but now we have plastic packaging which is causing toxicity. We are now being exposed to more styrene, dioxins, xylenes and dichlorobenzenes than ever before.

On top of that, we are exposing ourselves to foods that are creating a leaky gut such as gluten, dairy and a whole host of other food intolerances. This leaky gut is then leading to autoimmune conditions and nutrient deficiencies caused by malabsorption.

We have a continuous array of detox products coming on the market, targeting one organ at a time. We have liver cleanses, we have digestive cleanses and we even have ones specifically targeted towards the kidneys.

But we are really missing the point here. In order to detoxify properly we need to heal the body as a whole. Water fasting is a great way to do this as it gives the digestive system a break and uses the energy that would be normally sent for digestion to instead heal other issues within the body.

Q10. Can I exercise when I am fasting?

Generally I do not recommend heavy exercise when you are fasting.

However, I go by the principle that you need to figure out what works for you. I have heard of some people that have managed to work out during fasting while others are too weak to do so.

For me, when I am water fasting I try to conserve energy and I just do as much meditative walking as I possibly can. Sometimes I can walk for 2-3 hours per day but I avoid any strenuous HIIT or Cardiovascular exercise.

In terms of Resistance training I do a few light weight bearing exercises every couple of days just to keep the muscles firing but I avoid anything like P90X or Turbo fire.

If you are doing a short water fast you could possibly do a heavy exercise session prior to your first meal – say after a couple of days but for longer sessions you need to conserve as much energy as you can for healing.

Also, another reason I do not recommend heavy exercise whilst water fasting is because heavy exercise is a stressor on the body and as cortisol is already slightly raised it is important to minimize any additional stressors.

Q11. Should I continue my medications when I am fasting?

As I am not a medical doctor I will not recommend either way but would instead recommend that you go and speak to your practitioner if you are on prescription medications and you are wanting to complete a water fast.

Some people say it is perfectly fine as long as the medications are able to be taken without food and others say to avoid it altogether. Also, sometimes your requirement for medications may change during the fast so the dosage may need to be changed. Therefore speak to your practitioner first about your options.

Q12. Can I fast if I am slim?

What is the reason for you wanting to fast? If you are slim and wanting to fast it is likely that you have some underlying condition you are wanting to treat. If that is the case, there are obviously tissues and organs that need to be healed and toxins that need to be eliminated. In this case it is perfectly fine for you to fast for a certain amount of time. For a slim person, I would generally recommend no longer than 10 days at a time.

Q13. How much weight will I lose when I am fasting?

I have absolutely no idea. How much weight you lose will depend on you individually. However, on average somebody may lose a pound a day, and even more if you have more weight to lose.

I have heard of people doing a water fast for 7 days and losing 20lbs. It just depends on your unique make up, how much sleep you get and how much stress you experience during the process as these all affect the fat burning process.

For instance, if you don't get enough sleep you may still have blood sugar levels equivalent to a diabetic, which means that even though you are not eating you are still halting the fat burning effect and increasing the likelihood that once you do start eating again the weight will be put back on very quickly.

Q14. Do I need to supplement electrolytes (salt, potassium) when fasting?

I would definitely recommend that if you are doing a longer fast you take electrolyte supplements. Electrolytes that I would specifically recommend include Salt/Sodium (Celtic Sea Salt), Potassium, Calcium, Phosphate and Magnesium. You are able to get these through supplements or just add some lemon and celtic sea salt into a glass of water and make your own electrolyte drink.

Q15. Can Children, Infants and the Elderly fast?

Although there are few reasons why children and infants need to do an extended fast, it is perfectly safe for them to fast for a small amount of time.

Have you ever noticed when your child is ill that they don't want to eat?

If so, that is their own bodies innate healing processes doing their job.

For infants, 2-3 days is the most I would recommend and then for children, 1-2 weeks is the longest I would recommend. Make sure that you keep a good eye on your child when they are doing it to make sure that they are not experiencing excessive dizziness and blurred vision.

If so, take them to the doctor for a checkup.

I know that my daughter often does a water fast for a couple of days with me and she reports amazing energy and increased productivity at school. It is important that your child is not resisting it but if they do show an interest in it then there is no reason to be afraid.

As for the elderly, there is absolutely no reason that they cannot do a full water fast, just like any other adult does. The only thing you would need to watch out for is the medications they are on.

Q16. Are enemas necessary during a fast?

No, enemas are absolutely not necessary during a fast. In fact, Dr Joel Fuhrman and Herbert Shelton (both experts in the field of fasting) recommend that you leave the bowels alone during this period.

It is completely normal to not have a bowel movement during this time as you are not consuming foods.

However, it is often beneficial to take a laxative about a day before you begin your fast so that you may empty your bowels and then one right after to eliminate anything that has been sitting there.

Chapter 16 – Other Fasting Protocols

In this section I have listed three other fasting protocols which I believe can be beneficial in the whole healing process. Now I know you are probably wondering why I haven't added juice fasting into the mix and I am going to tell you right now.

Juice fasting to me is a great way to increase your blood sugar levels, especially as most people that do a juice fast need to have some fruit in it as well as vegetables to make it palatable.

Although it does give your digestive system a little bit of a break, the rapid rise in blood sugar levels are also going to increase inflammation and make the healing process a lot more difficult.

Therefore, the three fasts I am going to discuss include:

- Intermittent Fasting;
- Bone Broth Fasting; and
- Dry Fasting

Although I believe water fasting is the way to go in terms of healing I do believe that these other 3 methods also have their place too.

Intermittent Fasting

Intermittent Fasting is a period of not eating. Some people schedule this intermittent fast (as shown in the different types of intermittent fasting protocols shown below) and others just go by their level of hunger or by how it fits into their lifestyle.

Intermittent Fasting is not a diet but a schedule that is used to accelerate fat loss and muscle growth compared to traditional eating schedules.

Calorie Restriction versus Intermittent Fasting

If you have been listening to the news for the last few years or watching shows like Dr Oz, you will have heard about the importance of Calorie Restriction and its effect on longevity. Calorie Restriction is a reduction of at least 30% of your calories below your maintenance level, which through numerous research studies has been shown to increase longevity and reduce the risk of age related illnesses.

However there are a couple of issues regarding calorie restriction that I must point out.

Firstly, it can be very difficult to adhere to, unless you are following a lower carb higher fat satiating diet. This plan is naturally satiating and will therefore create a calorie restriction all on its own, without you needing to count calories, as long as your protein levels are not too high.

But, if you are trying to do calorie restriction by following a standard diet you may find it rather difficult as you are required to count your calories on a daily basis, you are restricted with what you can eat and the constant bombardment of carbohydrates can cause you to be even hungrier.

Secondly, if you drop your calories too low (especially if you are not consuming sufficient micronutrients) you may find that your body perceives itself as starving. Ensure that you are getting at least 1200 calories per day to avoid this happening.

Thirdly, calorie restriction can take weeks or months to achieve the same benefits that day long fasting is able to achieve.

So, instead of restricting your calories on a daily basis and experiencing that hunger that you do, how about mimicking the effects of calorie restriction but without the need to count calories?

That is where intermittent fasting comes in. Although there is not as much research out there on fasting as opposed to caloric restriction it works on the same principle, with even more added benefits.

Let's think about it for a moment. If we are only able to eat within an 8 hour window then obviously you are going to eat fewer calories anyway. Naturally your body can only eat so much at a time. Yes, I know what you are thinking... What about all the people that gorge themselves on food at the end of the day in their 8 hour window.

Wouldn't it be better to spread that food out over the day? What I have to say to that is "not necessarily, but it depends".

I know this book is written on fasting and the benefits of such but I need to point out that fasting is not for everybody and you need to figure it out for yourself. If reducing your calories throughout the day makes more sense to you and you feel better doing that, then go right ahead and do that. If you don't mind counting calories to make sure that you are in that 30% below calorie limit then that is no problem.

However, the benefit of taking that window of fasting, especially if you fast right through breakfast up until about 2pm or 3pm is that you are in a ketotic state that whole time, burning fat and going through a process of autophagy – which doesn't happen as long as you are in a constant state of digestion.

However, I will leave it up to you to decide which is right for you...

One thing that I must point out though before I wrap up this section is that no matter what you choose you must ensure that you are getting enough micronutrients to sustain a healthy body.

Even if you are intermittently fasting, deciding to eat cheerios and kit kats at the end of the day, alongside that entire pizza is not the way to take full advantage of the effects of the fast. Try to still keep your evening meal as low carb as possible so as to optimize your burning of fat.

If you have no weight issues and you are doing this purely for health benefits then more carbs may be able to be implemented, just try to keep them as natural and healthy as possible (with the odd treat thrown in if you must). After all, life is for living and so the last thing that I want is for you to feel miserable. All I can say is "Don't go crazy on the sugars".

The results of calorie restriction and ageing are varied, with some indicating that they see no effects and others indicating that there is benefit regarding increasing the lifespan of monkeys and rodents (see research studies below). However, there are also indications that calorie restriction may delay or prevent the onset of certain lifestyle diseases.

The dangers of calorie restriction is that consistent restriction in calories can lead to changes in metabolic rate. However, fasting up to 24 hours in humans does not seem to adversely affect blood glucose levels, muscle mass or cognition.

Types of Intermittent Fasting

There are a multitude of different intermittent fasting regimes out there that you are able to choose from if Intermittent Fasting is the way you are wanting to go...

Protocol #1 - Lean Gains by Martin Berkhan

This method encourages fasting for 16 hours and then consume 3 meals over the next 8 hour period. If you work out during the day, you exercise before your first meal of the day to make sure you are consuming sufficient protein post-workout. He also recommends taking 10g branched chain amino acids about 15 minutes before your workout so as to minimize muscle breakdown during the workout.

They have found that although men typically do well on this plan, women often need a larger eating window and a small 14 hour fast.

Protocol #2 - The Warrior Diet

This method promotes one large healthy meal per day with the option to eat small snacks of raw fruits and veggies, fresh juice and a few servings of protein. It involves low calorie eating over a 20 hour period with a 4 hour period where you eat a normal meal.

Although it has been shown to be effective with fat loss (shown below), over the 8 week period with only 1 meal per day they found that the hunger steadily increased as the appetite hormone did not acclimate.

Protocol #3 - Alternate Day Fasting

As the name suggests, this is when you eat normally for 24 hours and then eat low calorie for 24 hours. Although this is a protocol that is often used when researching intermittent fasting in animals, studies of this kind have not been done in humans.

Protocol #4 - Eat Stop Eat by Brad Pilon.

This is a fast that is done for 24 hours and can be started at any time of the day and at different frequencies but is generally not done more than 1-2 times per week.

Steps to Start Your Own Intermittent Fast

Dial in your nutrition

It is very important that prior to starting your own fast you make sure you are eating nutritiously. Eliminate grains, legumes, sugar and vegetable oils and if you are needing to lose fat, then reduce your carbohydrate levels and make sure you are consuming sufficient fats.

Become a fat burner by following a ketogenic diet as that will eliminate any hunger you may feel from being a sugar burner.

Get quality sleep

As mentioned previously if you are sleep deprived it is not a good time to begin a fast. Sleep deprivation is a stressor on the body and as fasting can also be a stressor you must make sure that your sleep is quality.

Reduce stress levels

If you are suffering from adrenal exhaustion or you are overly stressed, make sure you get a handle on it. You can either do this by practicing meditation, yoga or a multitude of other techniques.

Figure out what type of Intermittent Fasting you are interested in.

Choose from any of the plans mentioned above or create your own. The main thing you need to take into account with intermittent fasting is making sure that you give your body a certain amount of time without eating for it to be effective (at least 12 hours).

There have been many people who practice an intermittent fast and then in their eating window they eat whatever they like.

Although this works for some I believe in practicing Intermittent Fasting for health, which means making sure that even the food within that window is of good quality and nutritious for the body. As you are already a fat burner, any calories burnt during the fast will come from fat and not from sugar.

If you want to keep your fat burning capabilities up, make sure that you are also trying to minimize carbohydrates when you are eating.

However, you could always try it with higher carbs and lower carbs and see which one works best for you.

Implement exercise into your day

Making sure that you keep up your exercise whilst fasting is important as it will allow you to burn even more fat. If you are using the most popular type of fast which is the 16 x 8 Lean Gains formula, then fasting between 10pm at night and 2pm the next day is a great way of doing this.

Complete your resistance training or HIIT training in a fasted state and then eat your first meal about ½ hour to an hour after the training. Therefore, if you eat your first meal at 2pm, try to do your training between 12pm and 1pm.

Bone Broth Fasting

What is Bone Broth Fasting?

Bone Broth is one of the most amazing "Real Foods" you can ever consume. It is the reason that your mum or your grandma (in my case) used to make you hot chicken soup when you were feeling under the weather.

Bone Broth has so many amazing properties that help to heal your gut and boost your immune system and can be useful during a period of fasting so as to preserve muscle mass.

Therefore unlike with water fasting you will still be able to exercise on this plan without being too concerned about muscle loss. However, if you read Chapter 10 you will know that although fasting creates some minimal muscle loss, it is not significant.

Bone Broth Fasting is a process where you abstain from any foods or liquids except for water and bone broth. To understand how this type of fasting is going to benefit you, all you need to do is look at the benefits of water fasting with the following additional benefits of Bone Broth...

What are the Benefits of Bone Broth?

Bone broth has many amazing benefits, including:

- It contains a high amount of glycine which provides multiple benefits of its own:
- It limits or prevents the breakdown of protein tissue (i.e. muscle);
- It is necessary for the detoxification of chemicals, which is why it is so beneficial when fasting;
- It is an Inhibitory Neurotransmitter which helps to improve sleep, boost memory and boost performance.
- It is full of minerals.
- It is high in Collagen, Gelatin, Proline, Glutamine and Glycosaminoglycans, which has been shown to enhance digestion and heal the gut.
- It makes skin supple by supplying your body with all the tools it needs to support itself, in particular collagen.

Making a Good Bone Broth

When selecting the bones for your bone broth it is important to use a variety of different types of bones, due to the fact that different marrow bones contain different types of marrow, such as yellow marrow or red marrow.

On top of this make sure you are getting the bones from the best source possible – preferably grass fed if it is beef and free range if it is poultry.

To make the broth, do the following:

- Place your bones in the oven and roast them for about 15 minutes at 200 degrees Celsius.
- Take the bones out and place them in a large stock pot and cover with filtered water.
- Add 2 tbsp. organic apple cider vinegar to the water prior to cooking as this will help pull the important nutrients out of the bones.
- Make sure the stock pot is filled with filtered water and put on the stove to boil. Leave plenty of room for the water to boil.
- Heat it slowly and bring the water to a boil. Once it has boiled I like to transfer it to a slow cooker and place it on low. This means I don't need to keep an eye on the stove.
- Cook chicken bones for anywhere from 6 to 48 hours and beef bones for anywhere from 12 to 72 hours.
- After cooking the broth will cool and a layer of fat will harden on the top. This layer is very important as it protects the broth underneath. Discard this layer when you are about to eat it.
- Consume this broth within 3 days or freeze for later use. Sip on this broth throughout the day, especially after exercise.

Dry Fasting

A dry fast is an absolute fast where you abstain from all water and all food. This type of fast is predominantly done for religious purposes or for quick detoxification. Although there has been a lot written up by the Russians on Dry Fasting, there is very little out there in the English Language.

In fact I could not find one single research study on dry fasting. This is the most intense of any of the fasting methods and is one that should only be done AFTER using the other fasting methods for at least 6 months. Do NOT go into a dry fast on its own without the correct preparation.

There are two different types of dry fasts:

Hard Dry Fast

With this type of fast, the faster is not allowed to have any water touch their bodies, such as no washing dishes, no taking baths, no taking showers and no brushing teeth.

Soft Dry Fast

With this type of fast, the faster is allowed to have water touch their bodies.

Prepare for a Dry Fast

As a Dry Fast is the most intensive type of fast you can do it is incredibly important for you to prepare for it properly.

Find an area where the air is fresh, moist and pure so that the moisture from the air may be absorbed through the skin.

Start off by completing water fasts for at least 6 months first before attempting a dry fast. Prior to starting a dry fast, I would recommend that you are able to water fast for at least 10 days without any issues.

How Do I Do A Dry Fast?

Start by doing a 36 hour dry fast, once a week, and then gradually increase the length of the fast.

Complete the dry fast for up to 3 days without medical supervision.

Cascade dry fast where you fast for one day and then eat for one day, fast for two days and eat for two days and then keep going. Dr Filonov (Russian Doctor) has found this to be a very safe way of doing a dry fast.

Do not do the dry fast for any longer than 12 days at a time, even under the supervision of a practitioner. 3 Days is optimal.

Avoid intense exercise when participating in a dry fast.

Avoid sun/heat during this period.

How Do You Exit A Dry Fast?

How you exit the dry fast is incredibly important, otherwise you could really harm yourself. It is important to drink 2 liters of pure water very slowly, holding each sip up to your mouth for as long as you can over a 2 hour period.

After this, it is recommended to reintroduce soft foods and liquids like bone broth, soups, smoothies etc. before reintroducing solid foods as it is important to allow your digestive system to gradually wean into it.

It is very important to rehydrate yourself by making sure you drink water slowly but consistently over a 12 hour period and possibly even integrate some coconut water into the mix which is very useful at rehydrating.

However, do not use pure coconut water as it can cause headaches and migraines if used in such large quantities. Try diluting it 3:1 (water : coconut water).

Dry Fasting Versus Water Fasting

Dry Fasting is a step up from water fasting and provides many benefits that are not seen in the water fasting:

Detoxification effects happen even quicker. With a water fast you will find that the toxins are removed through the bowels, skin, liver, kidneys and urine, but with dry fasting each cell is turned into an incinerator and the toxins are burned within the cells.

This means no body odor or bad breath.

Each day of a dry fast is seen to be equivalent to 3 days of a water fast.

That means that a 10 day dry fast is equivalent to a 30 day water fast.

You lose less muscle mass and more body fat with a dry fast than a water fast.

Who Shouldn't Do A Dry Water Fast?

There are a number of conditions where Dry Fasting is contraindicated, such as:

- Malignant Tumors;
- Blood Conditions;
- Tuberculosis;
- Hyperthyroidism;
- Endocrine Diseases;
- Cirrhosis of the Liver;
- Heart Arrhythmia;
- Circulatory Failure;
- Underweight;
- Pregnancy and Lactation;
- Being Under 14;
- Being Over 70.

Chapter 17 – Conclusion

I hope that you have received all the information you need from this book to start you on your own journey with water fasting. No matter whether you are trying to lose body fat or heal an illness water fasting could be a solution for you.

Throughout the book you will notice that I mentioned entering ketosis or following the ketogenic diet. If you are not quite sure how to get started on your own keto plan then I have written a couple of books that you may find useful:

Understanding Keto - Beginners Guide to the Ketogenic Diet;
Keto Blocks - 40 Reasons why you may be plateauing on your Keto Diet.

Also, if you sign up for the mailing list by going to http://www.lowcarbketoliving.com/freelist then you will receive additional content that will help you on your own journey towards health.

Cheers,

Naturopath Jen

Chapter 18 – References - Scientific

1. Alirezaei, M et al, "Short Term Fasting Induces profound Neuronal Autophagy", Autophagy 2010.

2. Walsh JJ et al, "Fasting and Exercise differentially regulate BDNF mRNA expression in human skeletal cells", Applied Physiology, Nutrition and Metabolism, 2015.

3. Newport MT et al, "A new way to produce hyperketonemia: use of ketone ester in a case of Alzheimers Disease", Alzheimers and Dementia, 2015.

4. Singh R et al, "Late-onset intermittent fasting dietary restriction as a potential intervention to retard age-associated brain function impairments in male rats", Age, 2012.

5. Wenzhen Duan et al, "Dietary restriction normalizes glucose metabolism and BDNF levels, slows disease progression, and increases survival in huntingtin mutant mice", PNAS, 2002.

6. Thiruma V Arumugam et al, "Age and Energy Intake Interact to Modify Cell Stress Pathways and Stroke Outcome", Ann Neurol, 2010.

7. Davis LM et al, "Fasting is neuroprotective following traumatic brain injury", Journal of Neuroscience Research, 2008.

8. Aksungar FB et al, "Interleukin 6, C-Reactive Protein and Biochemical Parameters during Prolonged Intermittent Fasting", Annals of Nutrition and Metabolism, 2007.

9. Felicien Karege et al, "Decreased serum brain-derived neurotrophic factor levels in major depressed patients", Psychiatry Research, 2002.

10. John M Freeman et al, "Seizures Decrease Rapidly After Fasting", JAMA Pediatrics, 1999.

11. KY Ho et al, "Fasting enhances growth hormone secretion and amplifies the complex rhythms of growth hormone secretion in man", Journal of Clinical Investigations, 1988.

12. Cameron JD et al, "Increased meal frequency does not promote greater weight loss in subjects who were prescribed an 8-week equi-energetic energy-restricted diet", British Journal of Nutrition, 2010.

13. Webber J et al, "The cardiovascular, metabolic and hormonal changes accompanying acute starvation in men and women", British Journal of Nutrition, 1994.

Chapter 19 – References - Websites
****

- http://nutritionstudies.org/fasting-effective-ancient-therapy-todays-health-concerns/
- http://www.collective-evolution.com/2014/10/22/fascinating-evidence-shows-why-water-fasting-could-be-one-of-the-healthiest-things-you-can-do/
- http://www.gaianstudies.org/articles4.htm
- https://www.nutritionalresearch.org/research/completed/Water-Fasting
- http://paleoleap.com/long-fasts/
- http://www.vanderbilt.edu/AnS/psychology/health_psychology/fast.htm
- http://www.healthy.net/scr/article.aspx?ID=1996
- http://www.healthy.net/Health/Article/Nutritional_Program_for_Fasting/1996/2
- http://www.healthy.net/Health/Article/Nutritional_Program_for_Fasting/1996/3
- http://www.healthy.net/Health/Article/Nutritional_Program_for_Fasting/1996/4
- http://www.healthy.net/Health/Article/Nutritional_Program_for_Fasting/1996/5
- http://www.healthy.net/Health/Article/Nutritional_Program_for_Fasting/1996/6
- http://www.healthy.net/scr/article.aspx?ID=1998
- http://www.healthy.net/Health/Article/Fasting_Mono_diets_and_Raw_Food_Days_and_Chelation_Therap/1998/2
- http://www.healthy.net/Health/Article/Fasting_Mono_diets_and_Raw_Food_Days_and_Chelation_Therap/1998/3
- http://www.healthy.net/Health/Article/Fasting_Mono_diets_and_Raw_Food_Days_and_Chelation_Therap/1998/4
- http://www.healthy.net/Health/Article/Fasting_Mono_diets_and_Raw_Food_Days_and_Chelation_Therap/1998/5
- http://www.healthy.net/Health/Article/Fasting_Mono_diets_and_Raw_Food_Days_and_Chelation_Therap/1998/6
- http://www.healthy.net/scr/article.aspx?ID=496
- http://www.healthy.net/Health/Article/Fasting_for_Health_and_as_an_Anti_Aging_Strategy/496/2

- http://www.healthy.net/Health/Article/Fasting_for_Health_and_as_an_Anti_Aging_Strategy/496/3
- http://www.healthy.net/Health/Article/Fasting_for_Health_and_as_an_Anti_Aging_Strategy/496/4
- http://www.healthy.net/Health/Article/Fasting_for_Health_and_as_an_Anti_Aging_Strategy/496/5
- http://www.healthy.net/Health/Article/Fasting_for_Health_and_as_an_Anti_Aging_Strategy/496/6
- http://www.healthy.net/scr/article.aspx?ID=1657
- http://www.healthy.net/Health/Article/Diet_Fasting_and_Reduction_of_Disease/1657/2
- http://www.healthy.net/Health/Article/Diet_Fasting_and_Reduction_of_Disease/1657/3
- http://www.cru.org/train-and-grow/devotional-life/7-steps-to-fasting.html
- http://www.cru.org/train-and-grow/devotional-life/7-steps-to-fasting.2.html
- http://www.cru.org/train-and-grow/devotional-life/7-steps-to-fasting.3.html
- http://www.cru.org/train-and-grow/devotional-life/7-steps-to-fasting.4.html
- http://www.healthpromoting.com/clinic-services/health-services/why-undergo-fast
- http://www.healthpromoting.com/water-fasting/who-benefits-fasting
- https://www.healthscience.org/education/fasting/fasting-research
- https://news.usc.edu/63669/fasting-triggers-stem-cell-regeneration-of-damaged-old-immune-system/
- http://www.ncbi.nlm.nih.gov/pubmed/11416824
- http://www.telegraph.co.uk/news/uknews/10878625/Fasting-for-three-days-can-regenerate-entire-immune-system-study-finds.html
- http://www.sciencedaily.com/releases/2011/04/110403090259.htm
- http://www.curezone.org/forums/am.asp?i=1968737
- http://www.medicalnewstoday.com/articles/277860.php
- http://www.livescience.com/48888-intermittent-fasting-benefits-weight-loss.html
- http://www.scientificamerican.com/article/how-intermittent-fasting-might-help-you-live-longer-healthier-life/

- http://easacademy.org/trainer-resources/article/intermittent-fasting
- http://www.marksdailyapple.com/fasting-brain-function/
- http://www.marksdailyapple.com/fasting-weight-loss/#axzz3dganKOs5
- http://www.marksdailyapple.com/fasting-cancer/
- http://www.marksdailyapple.com/fasting-cancer/
- http://www.marksdailyapple.com/fasting-cancer/
- http://www.marksdailyapple.com/fasting-questions-answers/#axzz3dganKOs5
- http://www.marksdailyapple.com/women-and-intermittent-fasting/#axzz3dganKOs5
- http://www.tylertolman.com/health-articles/water-fasting-benefits-detox-cleanse/
- http://orthodoxinfo.com/praxis/father-seraphim-rose-fasting-rules.aspx
- http://hinduismfacts.org/fasting-in-hinduism/
- https://en.wikipedia.org/?title=Fasting#Judaism
- http://www.whatdomormonsbelieve.com/2009/02/fasting/
- https://en.wikipedia.org/?title=Ramadan
- http://chestofbooks.com/health/Isabelle-A-Moser/How-and-When-to-Be-Your-Own-Doctor/Common-Fasting-Complaints-And-Discomforts.html#.VYnjw_mqqko
- http://www.curezone.org/forums/am.asp?i=1161285
- http://www.gaiamtv.com/article/how-fasting-can-increase-your-awareness
- http://www.howtofast.net/water-fasting.html
- http://www.allaboutfasting.com/breaking-a-fast.html
- https://dorothysager.wordpress.com/2012/10/05/am-i-losing-muscle-during-a-water-fast/
- http://waterfastingblog.com/tag/deficiencies
- http://www.cosozo.com/article/10-common-myths-about-fasting
- http://www.quickfasting.com/more_q_a_s.html
- http://bradpilon.com/weight-loss/intermittent-fasting-and-depression-an-inflammation-link/

Made in the USA
Middletown, DE
04 September 2016